CONQUERING DIABETES

A proven strategy to reverse insulin resistance, optimize blood sugar level and improve your overall health.

By JOMUEL SMITH | Copyright @ 2023

CONTENT

Introduction

Chapter 1: Conquering Diabetes Approach

Chapter 2: Getting Started with The Mastering Diabetes Method

Chapter 3: What Really Causes Insulin Resistance?

Chapter 4: Your Carbohydrate Master Class

Chapter 5: A comparison of the long- and short-term effects of the ketogenic diet with the low-fat plant-based whole-food diet

Chapter 6: All Fat Is Not Created Equal

Chapter 7: Contributing Culprit: Animal Foods.

Chapter 8: Learning About Your New Needs: Managing Oral Medications and Diagnostic Blood Tests

Chapter 9: Starting Strong: Breakfast

Chapter 10: Gaining Momentum: Launch

Chapter 11: Developing a Routine: Dinner

Chapter 12: Exercising for Maximum Insulin Sensitivity

Chapter 13: Intermittent Fasting for Insulin Sensitivity and Loss of Weight

Chapter 14: Meal Plans & Recipes

INTRODUCTION

Your visit to "Conquering Diabetes" is appreciated. We analyze the challenges of managing diabetes in this complete book using a mindful culinary approach. A complex understanding of diet and meal preparation is necessary for people with diabetes, a metabolic disorder that affects millions of people. Our goal is to arm you with the information and meal plans you need to acquire the skill of controlling blood sugar levels while enjoying scrumptious and healthy meals. This book provides a methodical way to creating a diabetes-friendly diet using science-based insights and useful culinary practices. This book will be your dependable travel companion on the road to effectively managing diabetes, whether you've recently been diagnosed or are looking to improve your eating habits. Prepare to set out on a culinary adventure that will enable you to take control of your health and enjoy the benefits of controlling your diabetes in the kitchen.

We shall explore diabetes' underlying causes and the critical role nutrition plays in its management in the chapters that follow. We'll explore the glycemic landscape while emphasizing how different foods affect blood sugar levels. With this information at your disposal, you'll be able to choose ingredients and plan meals with confidence.

There is something for you in our collection of recipes, which covers a wide range of tastes and preferences. Every dish, from filling breakfasts to gratifying dinners and everything in between, is painstakingly prepared to not only please your palate but also to support diabetes control objectives.

Additionally, we'll show you how to use cooking methods that maximize nutrient retention and improve flavors without endangering your health. You will learn the abilities necessary to prepare meals that strike the precise balance between flavor and blood sugar control through useful advice and detailed instructions.

This book will direct you toward a future of confident cooking and well-managed diabetes, regardless of whether you're navigating the early stages of the disease or looking to overhaul your culinary repertoire. As we learn how to master diabetes via the art of cooking, get ready to embark on a revolutionary culinary journey.

Knowledge really is power when it comes to managing diabetes. It is crucial to comprehend the intricate metabolic processes that control blood sugar levels. We will examine the science of diabetes, demystifying insulin resistance, carbohydrate metabolism, and the crucial function that macronutrients—carbohydrates, proteins, and fats—play in preserving glucose balance.

We'll go through a variety of delectable, diabetes-friendly dishes armed with this basic information. These dishes have been carefully chosen to establish a balance between flavor, dietary value, and glycemic index. Each recipe, which ranges from filling salads and hearty main courses to decadent desserts, is proof that treating diabetes does not mean giving up delicious food.

CHAPTER 1

CONQUERING DIABETES APPROACH

In our book, "Conquering Diabetes: A Logical Approach for Beginners," we set out to give you the information and resources you need to effectively manage diabetes from the outset. Understanding diabetes, a sophisticated metabolic condition, in its entirety is essential for navigating the road to optimum health.

Learn about the basics of diabetes, such as the kinds, the causes, and the processes that control blood sugar levels. With this knowledge, you'll be well-equipped to appropriately manage the illness.

We then discuss nutrition, which is crucial for managing diabetes. Learn how to control portions, measure carbohydrates, and use the glycemic index to keep your blood sugar levels consistent. Learn how to create a diet that is well-balanced, suited to your requirements, and places a focus on whole, unprocessed foods to enhance glycemic control.

Exercise is a crucial component as well. Discover how to incorporate a proper routine into your day and comprehend how exercise affects insulin sensitivity. A balanced diet and physical exercise regimen can improve blood sugar control and general quality of life.

Another important factor is medication management. Learn about different pharmaceuticals, how they function, and the best methods and times to take them. You have the power to collaborate with your healthcare team to improve your diabetes management strategy when you are aware of the medications that are being given to you.

In our topic on monitoring and periodic exams, we emphasize the need of self-monitoring, frequent medical evaluations, and keeping proactive communication with medical specialists. After that, you may make decisions based on knowledge that advances your health objectives.

Understanding diabetes, including its types, causes, and physiological systems that control blood sugar levels, should be your first step. You will find it simpler to understand the main ideas required for effective diabetes therapy once you have this factual basis in place.

This method's base is a thorough knowledge of diet, which is essential for controlling blood sugar levels. You may make a balanced meal plan that consists primarily of whole, unprocessed foods by comprehending the complexities of the glycemic index, carbohydrate counting, and portion control. You can maintain better glycemic control by eating sensibly.

The significance of effective drug management cannot be overstated. Learn about diabetes medications, including how they work, how to take them correctly, and any possible adverse effects. By being aware of the suggested treatments, you may collaborate with healthcare professionals to develop the best diabetes control plan.

Routine monitoring and exams break up this meticulous approach. By putting a focus on self-monitoring and sticking to routine medical checkups, you may encourage proactive interaction with your healthcare team. If you have access to verifiable information, you can make decisions that are in keeping with your health objectives.

Equally crucial is having a good grasp of medication management. Examine the specifics of diabetic medications, such as their mechanisms of action, suggested doses, and potential side effects. When you know how to give prescription drugs correctly, you may collaborate with healthcare professionals to maximize your diabetes management strategy. The value of regular observation and physical examinations cannot be overstated. To allow data-driven decision-making with your healthcare team, adopt a proactive approach by regularly monitoring your health and scheduling exams.

CHAPTER 2

GETTING STARTED WITH THE CONQUERING DIABETES METHOD

A well-organized and educational diabetic cookbook designed for beginners may be a crucial tool in tackling the issue of controlling diabetes, especially for people who are unfamiliar with the illness. This article looks into the principles of a cookbook (**CONQUERING DIABETES**) like this, highlighting the "Conquering Diabetes Method" and how it offers a reasonable strategy for managing diabetes.

1. Being aware of the Mastering Diabetes Technique

An organized method to managing diabetes that places a focus on a plant-based, low-fat, whole-food diet is known as the Mastering Diabetes Method. This approach seeks to maximize insulin sensitivity, which is important for managing diabetes. Whole grains, fruits, vegetables, and legumes make up the majority of the diet, while low-fat and processed carbs are minimized or completely avoided.

2. The Role of Diet in the Management of Diabetes

Because it directly affects blood sugar levels, diet is important for managing diabetes. The conquering Diabetes Method places a strong emphasis on the value of eating nutrient-dense, fiber-rich foods to lower insulin resistance and help regulate blood sugar levels. People can better control their diabetes and possibly lessen their need on medication by concentrating on complete, plant-based diets.

3. Creating a book for Diabetes for Beginners

Conquering Diabetic Method-based diabetic book for beginners should offer thorough instruction. It should include simple-to-follow meal plans, recipes, and instructional material to help readers comprehend the reasoning behind the diet recommendations. The book ought to explain how various meals affect blood sugar levels and why some diet decisions are advantageous for controlling diabetes.

4. Combining pragmatism with simplicity

In order for the book to be successful, simplicity and usefulness must come first. Recipes should make use of materials that are easily accessible, provide clear cooking directions, and place a priority on taste without sacrificing health objectives. Additionally, the cookbook need to provide guidance on meal planning, portion management, and appropriate food pairings to help new dieters establish a long-term eating schedule.

5. Enabling Novices to Take Charge

People are given the information and resources they need to control their diabetes by putting the Conquering Diabetes book for beginners. This method's rational approach and scientific backing provide people confidence in treating diabetes through dietary decisions. The book serves as an excellent place to start, pointing newcomers in the direction of a better, more balanced way of living.

6. Following evidence-based guidelines

The Conquering Diabetes book is based on ideas that have been proven effective in increasing glycemic control and insulin sensitivity. It avoids fad diets and places a focus on eating whole, low-fat plant-based meals. Since it is in line with tactics that have scientific backing, this rational approach is essential for novices and increases the authority and potency of the diabetic book.

7. Dispelling Nutritional Myths

Navigating a sea of nutritional information is one of the major challenges experienced by those who have just received a diabetes diagnosis. The Conquering diabetic book dispels persistent myths and misconceptions about nutrition and diabetes. It offers a basic and unambiguous viewpoint on nutrition, clearing up any doubt and promoting a reasoned knowledge of dietary options.

8. Dealing with Variability and Meal Planning

Meal planning and dietary variety are covered in a well-organized diabetic cookbook. It provides a wide variety of recipes appropriate for various meals, guaranteeing that people may maintain a satiating and nutrient-dense diet. The cookbook encourages diversity without straying from the logical principles of diabetes control by offering choices that are consistent with the Mastering Diabetes Method.

9. Promoting Long-Term Lifestyle Changes

A crucial component of managing diabetes is sustainability. The cookbook need to promote long-term, sustainable lifestyle improvements in addition to rapid effects. The Mastering Diabetes Method, which is based on a holistic view of health, encourages people to select an eating strategy they can stick with and apply to their regular lives in order to reap long-term advantages.

10. Stressing Education and Personal Effectiveness

Education should come first in a diabetic book based on the Conquering diabetic Method. It ought to make it apparent how different foods impact insulin sensitivity, blood sugar levels, and general health. The book gives people the knowledge they need to make wise decisions, improving self-efficacy and helping them to actively participate in controlling their diabetes.

11. Creating a Community of Support

A diabetic book for beginners should recognize the value of a caring environment. The Conquering Diabetes Method offers a forum for connecting with people who use a similar dietary strategy, encouraging interaction and the exchange of experiences, advice, and support. This sensation of belonging to a group supports the method's logical foundations and makes it easier to follow the recommended diet.

12. Monitoring Results and Changing Approaches

Monitoring results and making necessary adjustments to strategy are essential components of diabetes treatment. Beginners should follow the diabetic book's instructions for keeping track of their nutritional intake, blood sugar levels, and general wellbeing. By include this element, people may rationally evaluate how the Conquering Diabetes Method affects their health and make appropriate modifications.

13. Encouragement of Regular Exercise

Regular physical exercise is crucial to managing diabetes along with dietary decisions. The book should support a balanced strategy that incorporates exercise in addition to the conquering Diabetes Method. Giving advice on appropriate workouts and their advantages, it promotes a holistic lifestyle that combines food and exercise for the best possible health outcomes.

CHAPTER 3

WHAT REALLY CAUSES INSULIN RESISTANCE

The complicated physiological condition known as insulin resistance occurs when your body cells stop responding to the hormone insulin, which is essential for controlling your blood sugar levels. Obesity, lifestyle, and heredity are the underlying culprits. Although some people are genetically predisposed to insulin resistance, lifestyle choices dramatically worsen the condition.

Overconsumption of harmful fats, sweets, and refined carbs can cause weight gain and increased fat deposition, especially around muscles and liver. This extra body fat interferes with proper insulin signaling, particularly in the visceral region. Adipose tissue produces chemicals that reduce the efficiency of insulin.

Sedentary lives make the problem worse. The muscles' capacity to use glucose effectively is decreased by inactivity, needing greater insulin levels to promote glucose absorption. This overworked pancreas eventually produces less insulin, which worsens insulin resistance.

Chronic inflammation, which is frequently brought on by a poor diet, stress, or underlying medical issues, is important. Inflammation can disrupt your body's capacity to utilize insulin properly by interfering with insulin signaling pathways.

By concentrating on a balanced diet, frequent exercise, and stress management to reduce the risk and consequences of insulin resistance, you can make educated lifestyle decisions.

Insulin resistance can be exacerbated by a number of medical illnesses and drugs in addition to lifestyle choices. Insulin resistance is frequently associated to hormonal illnesses including polycystic ovarian syndrome (PCOS), as well as PCOS.

It's crucial to address chronic inflammation, which is typically as a result of a poor diet, stress, or underlying medical conditions. Inflammation interferes with insulin signaling pathways, which impairs the body's ability to use insulin as intended.

People may choose a healthy lifestyle by focusing on a balanced diet, regular exercise, and stress management to lower the risk and effects of insulin resistance.

In addition to lifestyle decisions, a variety of medical conditions and medications can make insulin resistance worse. Polycystic ovarian syndrome (PCOS) and other hormonal diseases are usually linked to insulin resistance. The hormonal anomalies linked to these illnesses make it challenging for the body to effectively regulate blood sugar.

The aging process can also lead to insulin resistance because of changes in body composition and a loss in physical activity that typically accompany aging. The body's ability to utilize glucose effectively decreases when muscle mass declines.

Finally, a person's predisposition to insulin resistance is greatly influenced by heredity. Certain genetic variations may affect how the body utilizes insulin and glucose. A family history of diabetes or insulin resistance increases a person's chance of developing the condition.

To effectively address and maintain insulin resistance, a complete approach that incorporates a healthy diet, consistent exercise, weight management, and medical aid for people with predispositions is required. People are better able to prevent insulin resistance and maintain overall health with this understanding.

Certainly. knowledge the molecular mechanisms of insulin resistance is crucial for a complete knowledge of this disease. Insulin resistance is primarily brought on by alterations to the insulin signaling pathway within cells.

In its natural state, insulin attaches to certain receptors on cell surfaces and sets off a series of signals that help cells absorb glucose from the circulation. Either the signaling pathways within the cells are messed up or the receptors become less sensitive in insulin resistance. As a result, the cell's capacity to efficiently absorb glucose is diminished, which raises blood sugar levels.

The insulin signaling pathway can sustain damage from cytokines and other inflammatory substances. Inflammation worsens insulin resistance because it hinders cells from functioning normally and interferes with insulin receptor activity.

Finally, insulin resistance manifests as a breakdown in the intricate signaling mechanisms that regulate the uptake of glucose by cells. The insulin signaling system is affected differently by a number of factors, including age, health problems, lifestyle choices, and genetic predisposition. The management of these factors requires a multifaceted approach in order to be effective.

CHAPTER 4

A MASTER CLASS IN CARBOHYDRATES

In the context of human nutrition, carbohydrates—often referred to as the body's main source of energy—represent a varied and crucial class of biomolecules. These organic substances are made up of carbon, hydrogen, and oxygen atoms that are grouped in various ways to provide a wide range of structures and functions essential for maintaining life.

Carbohydrates come in a wide variety of forms, from straightforward sugars like glucose and fructose to intricate polysaccharides like cellulose and glycogen. This variety results from the many ways that monosaccharide units are linked together, as well as from the length of the whole chain.

Monosaccharides: The Foundation:

The basic building blocks of carbohydrates are single sugar molecules, or monosaccharides. Among the most prevalent monosaccharides are glucose, fructose, and galactose, which operate as vital energy sources and take part in cellular operations.

Disaccharides and Polysaccharides:

Disaccharides are produced when two monosaccharides condense, such as sucrose (table sugar) and lactose (found in milk). Contrarily, polysaccharides are lengthy chains of monosaccharides that provide important functions including energy storage (such as starch in plants and glycogen in animals) and structural support (such as cellulose in plant cell walls).

Carbohydrates are the main source of energy in the human diet, which has a significant impact on metabolism. After being digested, complex carbohydrates are converted to glucose, which is subsequently used as fuel by cells. A hormone called insulin controls glucose levels, guaranteeing a sufficient and consistent supply to the cells.

Natural Cleanser: Fiber

For the preservation of digestive health, dietary fiber, a kind of carbohydrate primarily found in plants, is essential. It facilitates digestion, controls bowel motions, and may even lower the risk of chronic illnesses like diabetes and heart disease.

Impact of Glycemic Index on Blood Sugar

The glycemic index (GI) calculates how rapidly foods high in carbohydrates elevate blood sugar levels. Understanding the GI enables people to choose the right amount of carbs to take, which is crucial for those who are managing illnesses like diabetes.

Achieving a Balanced Carbohydrate consumption:

Opting for complex, unprocessed carbs over simple sweets and processed meals can help you maintain a healthy carbohydrate consumption. This option offers long-lasting energy, encourages satiety, and enhances general wellbeing.

Exercise and Carbohydrates:

Carbohydrates are essential for improving athletic performance. Consuming carbs before working out refills glycogen reserves, giving the body the energy and endurance it needs. For endurance athletes and anyone who train out for an extended period of time or intensely, this exercise is very crucial.

Carbohydrates and Cultural Significance:

Carbohydrates play a significant role in the diets of many people throughout the globe. Foods heavy in carbohydrates, such as rice, wheat, maize, potatoes, and others, have cultural, historical, and social value that showcases the diversity of culinary practices across the world.

The main fuel for the brain, glucose, supports mental processes including memory and focus. Carbohydrates and Brain Function in order to give the brain a consistent and suitable supply of glucose for maximum function, a balanced diet of carbs is required.

The kind and amount of carbohydrates consumed matter, even though they are essential for optimal health. Increased weight, obesity, type 2 diabetes, and other metabolic diseases can result from consuming too many refined carbs and added sugars. Instead, maintaining excellent health requires adding healthy grains, fruits, vegetables, and legumes to your diet.

Inducing ketosis, a metabolic state in which the body burns fat for energy instead of carbohydrates, is the goal of both low-carb and ketogenic diets.

These diets have much lower carbohydrate intake. These diets are frequently used to lose additional weight or address certain medical issues. However, particular strategies and careful attention are needed to manage their long-term health impacts.

According to the national dietary guidelines, a balanced diet should contain a range of macronutrients, including carbohydrates. These recommendations stress the need of selecting complete, unprocessed sources of carbohydrates and keeping an eye on total calorie intake in order to maintain a healthy, sustainable diet.

Finally, being aware of the nuances of carbohydrates and their variety of physiological functions enables us to make nutrient-dense dietary selections. To live a healthy and full life, we must balance our carbohydrate consumption, take into account their sources, and comprehend how they impact our metabolism and general health.

Carbohydrates are an intriguing and important class of macromolecules that provide the body energy, sustain structural elements, and improve general health. We may choose our food wisely for a healthier and more active life by being aware of the many forms of carbohydrates and how they affect the body.

CHAPTER 5

A COMPARISON OF THE LONG - AND SHORT-TERM EFFECTS OF THE KETOGENIC DIET WITH THE LOW-FAT PLANT-BASED WHOLE-FOOD DIET

The low-fat plant-based whole-food diet and the ketogenic diet are two different approaches to nutrition, and each has its own particular long and short-term impacts on the human body.

The main goals of the ketogenic diet are to reduce carbohydrate intake and to encourage high fat consumption, which results in the metabolic condition known as ketosis. Rapid weight reduction as a result of decreased water retention and early fat utilization are frequent short-term consequences. However, this diet's restriction might result in vitamin deficiency and constipation.

In contrast, the low-fat plant-based whole-food diet places a focus on a wide range of fruits, vegetables, whole grains, and legumes, as well as on consuming little to no fat. Improved digestion, more energy, and better glucose control are possible short-term impacts. However, when the digestive system adjusts to an increased fiber intake, switching to this diet may initially produce gastrointestinal discomfort.

Long-term weight loss and better cardiovascular health indicators may result from the ketogenic diet, although concerns have been raised about an increased risk of heart disease owing to high saturated fat intake. On the other hand, a low-fat plant-based, whole-foods diet has been shown to improve long-term weight control, lower the risk of chronic illnesses, and boost heart health.

Both diets have advantages and disadvantages, so selecting the best strategy requires careful evaluation of each person's unique health objectives, way of life, and dietary requirements. Regardless of the dietary strategy adopted, balancing macronutrients, consuming a variety of nutritious foods, and getting tailored advice from a healthcare provider are still essential.

1. *Weight reduction and Metabolic Effects:*

- **Ketogenic Diet:** When the body is in a state of ketosis, there is frequently noticeable short-term weight reduction. The durability of this weight reduction over the long term, however, is still a worry, and if carbohydrate intake is resumed, there is a considerable risk of weight gain.

- **Low-Fat Plant-Based Diet:** Although weight reduction may not occur as quickly as with the Ketogenic Diet in the short term, it frequently lasts longer. This diet's high fiber and low fat composition can support a healthy metabolism while helping to gradually lose extra weight.

2. *Nutritional Intake and shortages:*

- **Ketogenic Diet:** Due to the restricted dietary variety and exclusion of certain food categories including fruits, vegetables, and whole grains, the potential for nutritional shortages is substantial. To satisfy vitamin and mineral demands, monitoring and supplementation are frequently essential.

- **Low-Fat Plant-Based Diet:** Due to the wide variety of plant-based foods, this diet is typically high in fiber, important vitamins, and minerals. To guarantee optimal consumption of several minerals, such vitamin B12, iron, and omega-3 fatty acids, meticulous preparation is necessary.

3. *Cardiovascular Health:*

- **Ketogenic Diet:** While short-term impacts may indicate benefits in lipid profiles, long-term implications of high saturated fat intake on cholesterol levels and heart health raise concerns.

- **Low-Fat Plant-Based Diet:** Due to the low saturated fat content and high fiber intake, long-term adherence frequently results in lower cholesterol levels, decreased risk of heart disease, and better cardiovascular health.

4. *Sustainability and Lifestyle:*

- **Ketogenic Diet:** can be difficult to keep over the long run owing to its restrictions and associated side effects, such as the "keto flu Due" to social and practical challenges, it is typically less appropriate for long-term adherence.

- **Low-Fat Plant-Based Diet:** Due to its adaptability, range of dietary alternatives, and conformity with cultural and societal standards, it is frequently regarded as being more sustainable. It makes a wider variety of food options possible, which makes long-term maintenance simpler.

5.*potential health risk:*

- **Ketogenic diet:** risks include constipation, nutritional shortages, ketoacidosis (in severe instances), and probable long-term negative effects on liver and kidney function.

- **Low-Fat Plant-Based Diet:** The main risks are to maintaining appropriate nutritional intake, especially vitamin B12, iron, calcium, and omega-3 fatty acids.

6. Psychological Aspects and Mental Health:

- **Ketogenic Diet**: Due to ketosis, some people may initially feel enhanced attention and mental clarity. However, the rigidity of the diet may cause emotions of deprivation and social isolation, which over time may have an adverse effect on general mental health.

- **Low-Fat Plant-Based Diet:** The diversity and quantity of whole foods may develop a healthy connection with food and a long-term, well-balanced eating style. The emphasis on plant-based diets may be in line with moral and environmental principles and promote mental health.

7. Diabetes Management:

- **Ketogenic Diet:** Due to reduced carbohydrate intake, short-term effects may indicate improvements in blood sugar management. However, long-term effects on glycemic management and insulin sensitivity are still being studied and may differ from person to person.

- **Low-fat plant-based diets:** are generally advantageous for diabetics because they have an emphasis on whole, unprocessed foods and have high fiber levels that can help control blood sugar levels. It fits very nicely with dietary advice for controlling diabetes.

8. Cancer risk and inflammation

- **Ketogenic Diet:** Due to the diet's influence on insulin levels, several studies show potential anti-inflammatory benefits and a decreased risk of some forms of cancer. However, further study is needed to determine the long-term impact on cancer risk.

- **Low-Fat Plant-Based Diet:** According to research, eating a plant-based diet is linked to a decreased risk of some malignancies and inflammation since plant foods are rich in antioxidants and phytochemicals

Ideas to Think About and Advice:

- **Individualization:** It's important to adjust a diet to suit your needs, tastes, and medical issues. A tailored strategy is necessary for success since what works for one individual may not work for you.

- **Consultations with Experts:** To ensure a nutritionally balanced approach that matches individual needs, speaking with healthcare professionals—including registered dietitians—before making any dietary adjustments is strongly advised.

- **Long-Term Sustainability**: Stressing the need of a long-term, satisfying diet is essential for good health and effective adherence. Think of a balanced strategy that fits your tastes and way of life.

CHAPTER 6

ALL FAT IS NOT CREATED EQUAL

The adage "All fat is not created equal" emphasizes the critical distinction between various dietary fats and how they influence your body in the context of nutrition and human health. The three main types of fats are saturated, unsaturated (including monounsaturated and polyunsaturated fats), and trans fats.

Animal products and some tropical oils are common sources of saturated fats, which are normally solid at room temperature. raised levels of LDL cholesterol, sometimes referred to as "bad" cholesterol, have been related to an increased risk of heart disease and other health problems. Saturated fat consumption is another factor that has been connected to raised levels of LDL cholesterol.

On the other side, unsaturated fats are mostly found in plant-based oils, nuts, seeds, and fatty fish. These fats, which are frequently regarded as heart-healthy, can reduce LDL cholesterol levels when consumed in moderation. Monounsaturated fats from foods like avocados and olive oil, as well as omega-3 and omega-6 fatty acids, have been shown to considerably improve cardiovascular health and have other advantageous benefits, such as reducing inflammation.

The artificial process of hydrogenation, which transforms fluid oils into solid fats, produces trans fats. In processed foods, trans fats are usually present and pose major health risks. They can drop HDL cholesterol, or what is commonly known to as "good" cholesterol, while increasing LDL cholesterol, which is particularly detrimental to heart health. Trans fat consumption is advised to be reduced or eliminated totally by several health groups.

Understanding these variations is necessary to provide proper dietary advice. Balance your fat consumption and prioritize unsaturated fats over saturated and trans fats to maintain a healthy diet. It is essential to read food labels, choose natural sources of fat, and pay attention to the overall quantity of fat in your daily food intake in order to maintain maximum health and wellness.

The body also responds to different lipid types differently. Lipids are necessary, for instance, for the regulation of hormones, the absorption of fat-soluble vitamins (A, D, E, and K), and the long-term storage of energy. Your body's metabolic systems may digest various types of ingested fats in various ways depending on their chemical makeup.

Saturated fats have a straight molecular structure as a result of the single time that the carbon atoms are bonded together. Due to their structural rigidity, they are solid at room temperature. Conversely, the structure of unsaturated fats is kinked by one or more double bonds, which causes them to be liquid at ambient temperature. The way these fats interact with our systems is significantly affected by this ostensibly little change in chemical structure.

Saturated fats are linked to atherosclerosis and other cardiovascular disorders due to their propensity to build up in the body and arteries.

Omega-3 fatty acids and other polyunsaturated fats, on the other hand, are crucial for lowering inflammation and enhancing cardiovascular health. Omega-3 fatty acids are thought to boost brain function and lower the risk of chronic diseases. They are typically found in fatty fish, flaxseed, and walnuts.

Trans fats are produced by the process of hydrogenation, despite having double bonds. Their natural structure is altered throughout this process, giving them the appearance of synthetic materials to the body. Trans fats have harmful consequences on health, including an increased risk of coronary artery disease and type 2 diabetes, since the body is unable to properly metabolize them.

Making educated dietary selections requires knowledge of the key differences in the chemical make-up of various fats and their biological effects. A balanced diet that promotes unsaturated fats, contains a variety of whole foods, and sets limitations on saturated and trans fats can have a major influence on overall health and longevity. One needs to carefully monitor their fat consumption if they want to live a healthy lifestyle.

The complexity of fats is heightened by the roles they perform in the human body in addition to their chemical composition.
The critical roles that fats play in the formation of cell membranes, the encouragement of fat-soluble vitamin absorption, and their function as energy storage highlight the significance of fats in a balanced diet.

It is important to remember that the location of double bonds affects the unique characteristics of unsaturated lipids. Contrary to polyunsaturated fats, which have several double bonds, monounsaturated fats only have one. Double bonds make molecules more flexible and hasten vital metabolic processes. Omega-3 and omega-6 polyunsaturated fatty acids are referred to be "necessary" fatty acids since the body cannot generate them and must instead obtain them from food.

Lipids have effects on the environment and social spheres in addition to having an effect on health. When considerations like land usage, water use, greenhouse gas emissions, and biodiversity are taken into account, the production and consumption of various fats have various ecological footprints. When selecting a source of fat, choosing plant-based versus animal-based fats can help create a more sustainable and fair food system.

The distinction between different forms of fat is also essential due to dietary choices and objectives. The necessity to choose healthy fats to enhance performance and recovery is highlighted by the possibility that athletes and others who engage in high-intensity exercise may need to consume a little amount of additional fat to fuel their efforts. On the other hand, persons attempting to lose weight or improve their general health may benefit from a wiser and more balanced approach to fat consumption.

One of the foundational ideas of nutrition and wellbeing is the understanding that not all fats are created equally. It is essential to comprehend the many types of fats, their complex physiological processes, how they influence the environment, and how much of them is appropriate in light of a person's health goals. Understanding this complexity and taking a well-informed stance on dietary fat consumption are necessary for leading a nuanced and intentional nutritional lifestyle.

CHAPTER 7

CONTRIBUTING CULPRIT: ANIMAL FOOD

Diabetes is a widespread medical disorder that affects millions of people worldwide and necessitates careful food planning. A well-written cookbook (**CONQUERING DIABETES BOOK**) that is geared toward novices is one of the crucial aids in treating this condition. The importance of animal-based foods and their possible influence on the control of diabetes should be taken into account while embarking on this nutritional path.

Animal products including meat, dairy, and eggs have long been a mainstay of human meals. But a growing amount of research links their intake to a higher risk of getting diabetes and having it got worse. The logical analysis is based on how these goods' nutritional profiles.

First off, animal products are frequently high in saturated fats, which are known to affect insulin sensitivity, a key component of managing diabetes. Saturated fats may make it more difficult for insulin to efficiently control blood sugar levels, which may result in increased insulin resistance.

Second, the cholesterol content of these goods is frequently high. Because people like you with diabetes are more likely to have cardiovascular issues, elevated cholesterol levels are associated with an increased risk of atherosclerosis.

Additionally, animal-based diets typically lack fiber, a nutrient essential for maintaining healthy blood sugar levels. Fiber assists in reducing the rate at which sugar is absorbed, minimizing unexpected surges, and fostering more stable blood glucose levels. The dearth of fiber in animal meals has the potential to upset this delicate equilibrium.

Plant-based foods, on the other hand, provide a positive alternative. They usually have zero cholesterol and little saturated fat. Additionally, plant-based diets are high in fiber, complex carbs, and a number of important vitamins and minerals, all of which help with better diabetes management.

Meat, dairy products, and eggs are examples of animal foods, which are renowned for their high protein content and noteworthy nutritional profiles. However, their nutritional makeup also contains substances that may make it difficult to control blood sugar, which is crucial for those with diabetes.

The fact that animal meals frequently have significant quantities of saturated fats is one of the main issues. Scientific research repeatedly links consuming too much saturated fat to impaired insulin sensitivity, a condition frequently seen in people with diabetes. Saturated fats may hinder insulin's ability to effectively control blood glucose levels, thereby making the diabetes condition worse.

Furthermore, dietary cholesterol is mostly obtained from animal-based foods. The disease known as atherosclerosis, which is defined by the hardening and constriction of arteries, can be exacerbated by elevated cholesterol levels in the body. This becomes a significant factor to take into account for those with diabetes who already have a higher risk of cardiovascular problems.

In comparison, the nutritional profile of plant-based diets is better. They are a good option for diabetes treatment since they generally contain less cholesterol and saturated fat. Diets based on plants also frequently contain a lot of fiber, which is important for regulating blood sugar. Fiber helps to slow down the absorption of sugar, promote stable blood glucose levels, and lessen the likelihood of unexpected surges.

An analysis of animal-based meals and their function in this context is necessary for a cookbook designed for beginners who want to control their diabetes efficiently.

Furthermore, animal products are frequently high in cholesterol, a substance associated to a number of health problems, including heart disease. Since people with diabetes are already more likely to develop cardiovascular problems, it is wise to watch how much cholesterol they consume. Due to the intrinsic cholesterol level in animal-based foods, a diet rich in these foods may increase this risk.

However, plant-based meals offer a substitute that is often devoid of dietary cholesterol and lower in saturated fats. These foods frequently have high levels of fiber, a nutrient essential for controlling diabetes. Fiber helps to improve blood glucose management, slow down the absorption of sugar, and lessen the likelihood of unexpected blood sugar increases.

A careful approach to eating is essential when starting a path to manage diabetes. This trip calls for a thorough investigation of animal-based meals and their possible influence on diabetes control, which calls for a beginner-friendly cookbook.

Additionally, these items frequently provide as important dietary cholesterol sources. Maintaining healthy cholesterol levels is crucial for diabetics who already have a higher risk of cardiovascular problems. Consuming foods derived from animals may unintentionally raise cholesterol levels, therefore aggravating this risk.

CHAPTER 8

LEARNING ABOUT YOUR NEW NEEDS: MANAGING ORAL
MEDICATIONS AND DIAGNOSTIC BLOOD TESTS

Understanding the complexities of treating a chronic illness like diabetes is crucial in the field of health and wellbeing. An excellent resource on this path to better health is a diabetic book designed for beginners. This article explores the key components of such a cookbook, concentrating on managing oral medicines and diagnostic blood tests as a necessary groundwork for successful diabetic care.

1. Diabetes Understanding: The Basics

Understanding diabetes is crucial to start with. Elevated blood sugar levels caused by either insufficient insulin synthesis or inefficient insulin use by the body define diabetes. To keep blood sugar levels within a safe range, careful monitoring and lifestyle changes are necessary.

2. Dietary Factors in the Management of Diabetes

In managing diabetes, diet is essential. A diabetic cookbook offers thorough guidance on how to prepare meals that efficiently control blood sugar levels while also meeting nutritional needs. The glycemic index of foods, portion management, and emphasis on balanced meals can help people take control of their dietary choices.

3. An Overview of Oral Medicines

Understanding oral drugs is essential for those with diabetes who have just received a diagnosis. Oral medicines work to reduce blood sugar levels in a number of ways, including by increasing insulin production, decreasing gastrointestinal absorption of glucose, or increasing insulin sensitivity. A diabetic cookbook for beginners explains the varieties, dosages, and potential adverse effects of various drugs, enabling people to decide on their treatment strategy with knowledge.

4. The Value of Medication Compliance

Effective diabetes management depends on taking prescription drugs as directed. A diabetic cookbook not only offers delicious and diabetes-friendly dishes, but it also informs readers on the need of strictly adhering to medication regimens. In order to keep blood sugar levels within the desired range and avoid consequences related to uncontrolled diabetes, this adherence is crucial.

5. Integrating Diagnostic Blood Tests with Blood Glucose Monitoring

For the management of diabetes, diagnostic blood tests, such as blood glucose monitoring, are crucial. The cookbook explains the need of routine blood sugar monitoring to novices and how these tests offer important information about how well food choices and medication regimes work. Understanding blood glucose levels enables quick corrections to keep blood sugar levels steady.

6. Meal Preparation and Recipes: Combining Health and Flavor

An essential component of managing diabetes is meal planning, which is made easier by a cookbook for people with diabetes. It provides information on how to prepare tasty, healthy meals that are suitable for people with diabetes. The cookbook provides a selection of dishes that strike a balance between flavor and health by utilizing whole grains, lean meats, and lots of veggies while also taking into account portion sizes and carbohydrate levels.

7. The Key to Diabetes Nutrition: Managing Carbohydrates

Controlling carbohydrates is essential for blood sugar regulation. Understanding carbohydrates, their effect on blood sugar levels, and methods to keep tabs on and regulate carbohydrate intake are all covered in a diabetic cookbook for beginners. Individuals can maintain stable blood glucose levels and make the necessary dietary changes by following practical advice on measuring carbs and making educated meal decisions.

8. Lifestyle adjustments and physical exercise

Combining physical exercise into everyday life, along with dietary changes, considerably aids in managing diabetes. The cookbook offers more than just meals; it also provides information on the value of regular exercise and recommends doable physical activities. People are inspired to include exercise into their daily routine by knowledge of the benefits of an active lifestyle on controlling blood sugar and general wellbeing.

9. Tracking Your Progress: Maintaining a Health Journal

A useful tool for tracking development and seeing trends in blood sugar levels, food choices, medication adherence, and physical activity is keeping a health diary. Beginners with diabetes are encouraged by a diabetic cookbook to keep a health diary so they may track their progress, figure out what works best for them, and work efficiently with medical experts for individualized diabetes treatment.

10. Seeking Expert Advice and Support

Finally, a diabetic cookbook stresses the significance of consulting medical experts for advice. A qualified diabetes management plan should be established with the help of a certified dietitian, endocrinologist, or diabetes educator. The cookbook promotes a proactive and knowledgeable approach to diabetes treatment by educating readers on the importance of routine checkups and consultations.

11. Overcoming Obstacles and Coping Mechanisms

Living with diabetes comes with its own set of difficulties, such as psychological and emotional issues. A diabetic cookbook dives into coping mechanisms and approaches for fostering resilience to address the psychological effects of the illness. It places a strong emphasis on having a happy outlook, asking for help from others, and investigating mindfulness techniques to get over any potential emotional obstacles.

12. Educating Relatives and Other Supportive Groups

Diabetes management includes not only the diagnosed person but also their close relatives and support systems. The cookbook offers advice on how to inform family members and close friends about diabetes, ensuring that they are aware of the disease, its nutritional consequences, and the value of working together to create an atmosphere that is encouraging and conducive to good treatment.

13. Adopting a Lifestyle That Is Long-Term and Sustainable

The diabetic cookbook promotes establishing a sustainable lifestyle that is consistent with long-term health objectives in addition to urgent control. It underlines the significance of incorporating the knowledge gained from the cookbook into daily activities, cultivating long-lasting habits that contribute to general wellbeing and sustained treatment of diabetes.

14. Honoring Achievements and Progress

For motivation and morale, acknowledging accomplishments in controlling diabetes is essential. The cookbook exhorts readers to acknowledge and build upon all of their accomplishments, no matter how little they may be. This encouraging feedback supports retaining a proactive and resolute mentality in the face of difficulties.

CHAPTER 9

STARTING STRONG: BREAKFAST

Breakfast is a good way to start.

Breakfast, which is sometimes praised as the most significant meal of the day, is crucial in determining how one will approach their day. Because of the prolonged fasting period experienced while sleeping, the morning meal is a crucial chance to restore the body's energy reserves and jump-start metabolic processes. The body's circadian cycle is synchronized by this mechanism, which maximizes food uptake and utilization all day long.

A breakfast that is well-rounded largely includes a balance of the macronutrients carbs, protein, and fat. A steady release of energy may be obtained from carbohydrates, ideally complex ones like whole grains. Proteins boost satiety by assisting in muscle development and repair, whereas healthy fats support a number of body processes and help you feel full.

Fiber-rich foods, such as fruits, vegetables, and whole grains, can help with digestion, stabilize blood sugar levels, and promote a feeling of fullness, which helps keep you from overeating later in the day. This factor is crucial for those who want to efficiently manage their weight.

Additionally, breakfast gives you the chance to make sure you're getting enough of the vitamins and minerals that are needed for your general wellbeing. Breakfast may assist reach a larger range of nutrients, fostering a healthy body and mind by including several dietary groups.

Starting the day with a healthy breakfast has been related to greater concentration and improved cognitive performance in addition to the physical advantages. Students and professionals should pay particular attention to this since it enhances their morning productivity and performance.

The success of breakfast, however, depends on the caliber of the food choices selected. It's crucial to choose nutrient-dense, less processed meals over sweet, calorie-dense alternatives. Long-term, such decisions can reduce the risk of obesity, diabetes, and other metabolic diseases.

The "most important meal of the day," breakfast, offers an essential framework for daily activities. As the name suggests, it breaks the fast experienced when sleeping and kickstarts the body's metabolic process. In order to restore energy levels and create a metabolic baseline to sustain physical and mental activity throughout the day, it is crucial to consume nutrients at the beginning of the day.

Breakfast's primary purpose is to strategically deliver important nutrients. The body uses carbohydrates as its main source of energy, whether they are found in whole grains, fruits, or vegetables. They provide a consistent flow of energy when ingested in the morning, promoting a constant level of alertness and attention.

Another important breakfast ingredient is protein, which promotes muscle growth and repair while also making you feel fuller and less likely to overeat later. Lean protein sources, such eggs, yogurt, or almonds, should be included to make a well-rounded morning meal.

Although they should be ingested in moderation, fats are also essential. For the proper functioning of the brain, the control of hormones, and the absorption of fat-soluble vitamins, healthy fats like those found in nuts, seeds, and avocados are crucial. These can be included in the morning meal to promote satiety and general health.

Breakfast's impact on eating choices throughout the day is an important consideration. Beginning the day with a balanced breakfast reduces unhealthy snacking and impulsive food decisions, setting the stage for successful meals throughout the day. Additionally, it keeps blood sugar levels stable, avoiding sudden spikes and subsequent dumps that can impair concentration and productivity.

The practice of skipping breakfast is common in our fast-paced environment. But doing so

In conclusion, breakfast is the foundation of a well-structured day since it gives you the energy and nutrition you need to start your day. To maintain energy levels, support body processes, and improve cognitive function, it should include the right balance of carbs, proteins, and fats. Understanding this key function and choosing well-informed, healthful breakfast options can encourage a better lifestyle and enhanced wellbeing.

On the other hand, proteins promote muscle development and repair. Lean protein sources in breakfast promote satiety, which lowers the tendency to snack on harmful foods before the next meal. In this sense, plant-based proteins, dairy products, and eggs are all fantastic options.

Fats, which are sometimes misinterpreted, are crucial for a number of body processes, including hormone balance and brain functioning. Avocados, nuts, and seeds are abundant sources of good fats, and include them in breakfast helps to provide a balanced diet.

For a balanced breakfast, fiber-rich foods are just as important as macronutrients. Fiber helps with digestion, keeps you from getting constipated, and makes you feel fuller faster. Dietary fiber may be found in abundance in fruits, vegetables, and whole grains, which raises the meal's total nutritional value.

Having a healthy supper is crucial for controlling blood sugar levels and managing diabetes. These 10 recipes have been thoughtfully selected to satisfy diabetics' dietary needs without sacrificing flavor or nutritional value.

1. Vegetable omelet:
Egg whites are a low-fat protein source.
Increase your intake of high-fiber veggies like spinach, tomatoes, and bell peppers to help with satiety and blood sugar management.

2. The Greek Yogurt Stand:
To avoid extra sugar, choose plain, sugar-free Greek yogurt.

For antioxidants and a controlled glycemic impact, add fresh berries to the layer.

3. Breakfast Quinoa Bowl:

Quinoa can be used as a low-glycemic alternative to traditional cereals. Add nuts for protein and good fats that aid in a gradual release of energy.

4. Toast made with whole grain bread and avocado:

Avocados' monounsaturated fats aid with blood sugar regulation. Choose whole grain bread to provide yourself more fiber and to help your digestive system.

5. Treat with Chia Seeds:

Chia seeds are a fantastic source of omega-3 fatty acids and fiber. Blend with unsweetened almond milk and top with a few berries for a high-nutrient treat.

6. Turned-over potatoes:

Use sweet potatoes instead of regular potatoes if you want potatoes with a lower glycemic index. Use lean protein sources, such as turkey or chicken sausage, for a well-balanced supper.

7. Villa Cheese and Berries:

Cottage cheese provides protein without increasing blood sugar. Serve with fresh berries to amp up the antioxidant content and give a touch of sweetness.

8. Breakfast Burrito with Veggies:

Place black beans, sautéed vegetables, and scrambled eggs within a whole grain tortilla.

This combination offers a balanced consumption of fiber, protein, and complex carbohydrates.

9. Smoothie with bananas and almond butter:

Blend almond milk without sugar, small banana, and almond butter together.

The healthy fats in almond butter slow down the digestion of carbohydrates, which stabilizes blood sugar levels.

10. Salmon roll and avocado:

Roll avocado and smoked salmon in a whole grain wrap for a power boost of omega-3s.

This mixture provides essential minerals and supports heart health.

These breakfast recipes provide a holistic approach to diabetes treatment through nutrition by highlighting lean proteins, healthy fats, and fiber-rich carbohydrates. You can have a pleasant and diverse breakfast without compromising optimal blood sugar management by mixing these options.

CHAPTER 10

GAINING MOMENTUM: LAUNCH

If you have diabetes, you must carefully monitor your food and make smart decisions to keep your blood sugar levels within a safe range. A crucial tool for navigating this nutritional path is a diabetes cookbook designed for beginners, which offers helpful advice and delectable dishes.

Diabetes is a common chronic disease that affects millions of people worldwide and is marked by improper insulin production or usage. A well-organized cookbook may be a useful resource for individuals who have just been diagnosed with diabetes because proper diet is crucial to controlling the disease. We'll explore into the realm of a diabetes cookbook for beginners in this tutorial, highlighting its importance and the launch dishes that make it a valuable tool.

Here are some recipes for launch:

1. Stir-fried veggies with tofu in them:

Include a variety of colorful, non-starchy vegetables.

Use tofu as a source of protein to help manage your glycemic index.

2. Salmon baked with asparagus:

Because of its high omega-3 fatty acid content, salmon is heart-healthy.

Asparagus fiber has minimal impact on blood sugar levels.

3. Quinoa with black bean salad:

Quinoa is a complex carbohydrate with a low glycemic index.

Black beans offer a fiber-protein combination that supports sustained energy.

4. Grilled Chicken with Herbs and Lemon Infusion:

Lean protein like chicken aids in the preservation of muscle mass.

Lemon adds flavor; sugar or unhealthy fats don't.

5. Pizza topped with veggies and cauliflower:

Use a cauliflower base instead of standard pizza dough to reduce carbs.

Eat lots of colorful vegetables for essential nutrients.

6. Feta and spinach stuffing inside a chicken breast:

Spinach has a low carb level and a high iron concentration.

Feta delivers a blast of flavor without going overboard with the saturated fats.

7. Curry made with chickpeas and eggplant:

Eggplants are high in fiber and antioxidants.

Chickpeas contain protein and slowly released carbohydrates.

8. Cherry tomatoes with zucchini noodles coated in pesto:

Zucchini noodles are a low-carb substitute for pasta.

Pesto incorporates heart-healthy fats and tastes good too.

9. Vegetable and turkey skewers:

Turkey and other lean protein foods aid in blood sugar regulation.

Mix with colorful vegetables for a high-nutrient meal.

10. Spinach and mushroom omelets:

Eggs may include high-quality protein as well as other nutrients.

Mushrooms and spinach offer a low-calorie, high-fiber addition.

These recipes emphasize nutrient density, balance, and low glycemic index ingredients, according to dietary guidelines that are beneficial for managing diabetes.

These extra dishes highlight the breadth and originality that a diabetes cookbook for beginners may provide. This cookbook offers dishes to accommodate all tastes and dietary requirements, including robust main courses, light and refreshing salads, and even guilt-free desserts.

Tips for Using the Diabetes Cookbook Effectively:

1.Planning and preparing meals:

- Utilize the guidebook to organize your weekly menus and include a range of dishes to maintain a healthy diet.
- To make cooking easier on hectic days, prepare the ingredients in advance.

2.Carbohydrate counting and portion control:

- To properly control blood sugar levels, pay attention to the serving amounts stated in the cookbook and use portion control.
- To maintain a constant carb intake, a key component of managing diabetes, learn to count carbs.

3.Regular evaluation and modifications:

- Regularly check your blood glucose levels to learn how various foods influence your body.
- Utilize this knowledge to modify recipes and serving sizes in accordance with your body's reaction.

4.Consultation with a Medical Professional
- Consult a healthcare provider or a trained dietitian before making substantial dietary changes. They may offer individualized advice based on your unique requirements and objectives.

5.Keeping Current and Informed:
- Keep up with the most recent developments in diabetes treatment and nutrition to improve your knowledge and use the cookbook with confidence.

This book provides advice on leading a better lifestyle in addition to recipes. It's a first step toward improved diabetes management since it gives you the skills and information you need to eat delectable food and keep your blood sugar under control.

CHAPTER 11

DEVELOPING A ROUTINE: DINNER

To guarantee a well-balanced and pleasant dinner, it is wise to establish a systematic routine. The dining experience may be made more interesting by building a repertory of varied dishes. Let's look at a couple thorough recipes that may be used with this procedure.

1. Lemon Herb Chicken on the Grill with Roasted Vegetables:

For at least 30 minutes, marinate chicken breasts in a combination of lemon juice, minced garlic, extra virgin olive oil, and other herbs.

Cook the marinated chicken on the grill until it is thoroughly done and has a lovely char.

Serve alongside roasted veggies, such as sweet potatoes, zucchini, and bell peppers. Before roasting them in the oven till soft, toss them with olive oil, salt, and pepper.

2. Stir-Fry with vegetables:

Stir-fry a variety of bright veggies in a little sesame oil in a wok, including broccoli, bell peppers, carrots, and snap peas.

Combine a soy sauce, ginger, garlic, and a dash of honey sauce with tofu or chickpeas for protein.

For a balanced and healthy dinner, serve over quinoa or brown rice that has been steam-cooked.

Bolognese spaghetti

Cook onions, garlic, and minced beef (or a plant-based option) until browned.

Crushed tomatoes in a can, tomato paste, dried oregano, basil, and a dash of sugar should all be added.

Simmer the sauce until it thickens. Serve with grated Parmesan cheese or a vegan substitute on top of whole-wheat spaghetti.

3. A chickpea curry

In a pan, sauté chopped onions, garlic, and ginger. Turmeric, cumin, coriander, and curry powder should be added.

Add coconut milk and canned chickpeas by stirring. Simmer for a while to let the flavors mingle.

Serve this vegetarian curry with brown rice or naan for a filling meal.

Use a variety of these dishes for supper each night to keep meals interesting and nutrient-dense. Mealtime may be made simpler while still providing a variety of flavors and nutritional advantages by planning ahead, prepping food beforehand, and sticking to a regular evening schedule.

4. Bell Peppers Stuffed with Quinoa:

Bell peppers' tops are cut off, and the seeds and membranes are taken out. Following the directions on the box, prepare the quinoa and combine it with the spinach, black beans, sautéed onions, and garlic.

Bake the bell peppers until they are soft after stuffing them with the quinoa mixture. Add cheese or nutritional yeast on the top.

5. Eggplant Parmesan in a bake:

Cut into rounds, breadcrumb-coated, and baked until crisp and golden are eggplant rounds that have been egg-bathed.

The cooked eggplant, marinara sauce, and mozzarella cheese should be arranged in a baking dish.

Bake the cheese in the oven until it is bubbling and melted. Serve alongside pasta or a crisp salad.

soup made with veggies and lentils

Celery, carrots, and onions should all be cooked in a pot until they are soft. Mince the garlic and add it just after.

Including potatoes, carrots, spinach, and diced tomatoes, add the lentils, vegetable broth, and a variety of other vegetables.

Vegetables and lentils should be cooked until tender. Pick your preferred herbs, then season with salt and pepper.

6. Grilled chicken salad:

Chicken breasts that have been grilled include lean protein.

Include a variety of non-starchy vegetables, such tomatoes, cucumbers, and leafy greens.

For a healthy fat source, dress with vinegar and olive oil.

7. Baked Salmon with Asparagus:

Salmon is high in omega-3 fatty acids, which are beneficial to heart health.

Asparagus adds fiber and essential nutrients.

Use lemon and herbs to season without adding more sugar.

8. Turkey stir-fried with veggies:

Lean ground turkey without additional fat provides protein.

Consume a bounty of colorful, low-carb vegetables, such bell peppers and broccoli.

Use a little amount of low-sodium soy sauce for flavor.

9. Shrimp and cauliflower rice bowl:

Replace ordinary rice with cauliflower rice to reduce your carb intake.

Shrimp are one type of low protein source.

Add chopped vegetables, like bell peppers and zucchini.

10. Vegetable-Stuffed Quinoa Peppers:

Quinoa is one of the whole grains with a low glycemic index.

Stuff bell peppers with black beans, mixed vegetables, and quinoa.

Roast peppers until they are tender.

11. Parmesan made from plants:

Slice the eggplant thinly and bake it instead of frying it.

Top one layer with a heaping portion of marinara sauce and part-skim mozzarella.

Serve with sautéed spinach on the side for an added nutritional boost.

12. Chicken and Broccoli Casserole:

Combine the chopped chicken breast with the steamed broccoli.

Serve with a light, low-fat cream sauce.

Pour in enough cheese and breadcrumbs and bake until bubbly.

13. Zoodles (zucchini noodles) with carbonara:

Instead of using spaghetti, use zucchini noodles.

A carbonara sauce is made with eggs, Parmesan cheese, and lean turkey bacon.

Sauté the zoodles and combine them with the sauce for a low-carb option.

Lentil and vegetable soup:

Lentils are a good source of fiber and protein.

Add a variety of colorful vegetables for added nourishment.

Opt for a broth-based soup to keep the calories and carbs under control.

Grilled Tofu and Vegetable Skewers:

Tofu is a plant-based protein source.

Put a variety of low-carb vegetables on a skewer, such cherry tomatoes, bell peppers, and mushrooms.

Marinate in a simple mixture of olive oil and herbs before to grilling.

These recipes focus on nutrient density, realistic portion sizes, and a balance of macronutrients to help control diabetes without sacrificing flavor.

CHAPTER 12

EXERCISING FOR MAXIMUM INSULIN SENSITIVITY

"Sensitivity" refers to the body's responsiveness to the effects of insulin. Less insulin will be needed by a person who is insulin sensitive to reduce blood glucose levels than by a person who is not.

Exercise is one of your best tools in the fight against diabetes. Exercise is even more important for optimal insulin sensitivity than a well-balanced diet. This in-depth manual will provide you useful guidance for properly managing your diabetes as well as an understanding of the complex link between exercise and insulin sensitivity. Think of this as your "Diabetes book" for improving insulin sensitivity via physical activity.

Knowing About Insulin Sensitivity

The pancreas secretes the hormone insulin, which is essential for controlling blood sugar levels. It enables cells to absorb glucose and convert it into energy. One of the main symptoms of diabetes mellitus is elevated blood sugar, which is brought on by an accumulation of glucose in the bloodstream as a result of insulin-resistant cells. Therefore, increasing insulin sensitivity is essential for managing diabetes.

Reduced Body Fat: Exercise helps regulate weight by assisting in the loss of excess body fat. Insulin resistance is linked to it.

Dietary components: You should combine a well-balanced diet with your exercise regimen. Consume meals high in fiber, lean protein sources, healthy fats, and complex carbs. Because carbohydrates are necessary for the management of blood sugar, you should watch how much of them you eat.

When and how often: Reliability is essential. Three days a week, one should engage in at least 150 minutes of moderate-intensity aerobic exercise or 75 minutes of vigorous-intensity aerobic exercise. For optimal results, perform weight training activities two or more days a week.

Keep an eye on your blood sugar: It is important to carry out regular blood sugar assessments. This enables you to modify your workout routine as necessary and helps you understand how your body reacts to exercise.

Conversing with medical specialists: It is essential that you speak with your healthcare provider before starting a new fitness program. They might offer recommendations based on your particular requirements, making sure that your workout regimen complements your entire approach to managing diabetes.

Cardiovascular Exercise: During and after an activity, blood sugar levels can be lowered by engaging in aerobic or cardiovascular workouts such brisk walking, cycling, or running. They provide rapid glycemic control and are highly effective in raising insulin sensitivity. Combining steady-state and interval exercise may result in a complete blood sugar management strategy.

Resistance Training: Using resistance bands or lifting weights are examples of resistance workouts that aid in the development and maintenance of muscular mass. Because muscle cells respond so strongly to insulin, having more muscle enhances one's ability to digest glucose. Your body uses glucose more efficiently when you put on muscle, which makes you more sensitive to insulin.

Post-Exercise Window: Following physical activity, particularly strength training, there is a "window of opportunity" during which your muscles are more sensitive to glucose. For the purpose of replenishing glycogen reserves and fostering muscle regeneration, it's important to consume a balanced meal or snack that includes both protein and carbs during this time.

Observe Your Body: When exercising, become aware of the cues your body is sending you. It's critical that you halt and check your blood sugar levels if you encounter symptoms such as weakness, dizziness, or excessive perspiration. Having a fast-acting glucose supply (glucose gel or a few pills) on hand is essential in case you need to treat hypoglycemia, which is a low blood sugar caused by exercise.

Hydration: People with diabetes need to drink a sufficient amount of water. Dehydration can interfere with the body's capacity to use glucose and have an impact on blood sugar levels. To stay properly hydrated, make sure you drink water before to, during, and following any exercise.

Support and Accountability: Join a diabetic support group or find an exercise partner. Having a support network might aid in keeping you accountable and motivated to complete your workouts. You might talk to people who are traveling a similar path and exchange problems, wisdom, and advice.

Long-Term advantages: Although physical activity may have an immediate effect on blood sugar levels, it's important to keep in mind that regular exercise has as important long-term advantages, if not more. Regular exercise lowers the risk of complications from diabetes by promoting long-lasting improvements in insulin sensitivity and general health.

The key to managing diabetes is to exercise to improve insulin sensitivity. It improves general health, lowers insulin resistance, and helps control blood sugar levels. These are only a few of the short- and long-term advantages it provides. You may control your diabetes and have a better, more active life with a healthy diet, frequent monitoring under the supervision of medical specialists, and the correct kinds of activity. Recall that in order to fully benefit from your efforts, you must be persistent and consistent.

CHAPTER 13

INTERMITTENT FASTING FOR INSULIN SENSITIVITY AND LOSS OF WEIGHT

The dietary practice of intermittent fasting (IF) has generated a lot of attention since it may have benefits for improving insulin sensitivity and encouraging weight loss. This eating plan prioritizes mealtime management above emotional reasons and is grounded in reason and science.

Understanding How to Sporadically Fast:

Intermittent fasting is a pattern of eating that differs between periods when one is fasting and when one is not, as opposed to a specific diet. It makes suggestions for when to eat certain meals, not what they should be consumed. Popular IF methods include the 16/8 strategy, which is a 16-hour fast followed by an 8-hour window for eating, and the 5:2 methods, which is a two-day period of drastically decreased calorie consumption followed by five days of regular eating.

1. Insulin Sensitivity: Insulin is a hormone that facilitates the uptake of glucose by cells, hence regulating blood glucose levels. High blood sugar levels are a hallmark of type 2 diabetes, which develops as cells become less sensitive to the effects of insulin. Intermittent fasting may enhance insulin sensitivity in a number of ways.

2. Reduced caloric intake: IF typically results in a decrease in caloric consumption overall. The body using less energy during fasting may lead to improved insulin sensitivity.

3. Weight Loss: Individuals who are overweight may benefit from IF. IF weight reduction can significantly improve insulin sensitivity since excess body fat is associated with insulin resistance.

4. steady Blood Sugar Levels: By minimizing the frequent insulin spikes through improved blood sugar management, IF aids in the body's maintenance of a steadier metabolic state.

5. Enhanced Cellular Repair: During a fast, the body activates processes like as autophagy, which aid in the removal of damaged cells and encourage the growth of new, healthy ones. An increase in insulin sensitivity might result from this.

6. Weight Loss with Intermittent Fasting: Metabolism, hormonal control, and calorie balance are all important factors in weight reduction. IF is effective for controlling weight due to several mechanisms:

7. Diminished Caloric Intake: As mentioned earlier, IF often causes a decrease in overall caloric intake, which establishes the calorie deficit necessary for weight loss.

8. Fat Burning: When fasting, the body burns fat stores as fuel, which contributes to the loss of body fat.

9. Benefits for Metabolic Rate: IF has the potential to increase metabolic rate, which might lead to an increase in energy expenditure.

10. Appetite Control: For some people, intermittent fasting (IF) helps them control their appetite, so following a calorie-restricted diet may be simpler.

11. Hormonal Balance: IF has a positive impact on hormones like ghrelin and leptin that are related to hunger and fullness.

Ability to React to Insulin:

1. Better Glucose Control: Insulin fusion (IF) allows pancreatic beta cells to rest and renew when insulin production is lowered during fasting intervals. This might eventually lead to an increase in insulin sensitivity.

2. Inflammation Reduction: IF has been associated with a decrease in inflammation, particularly in adipose tissue. Reducing inflammation can aid in the reduction of insulin resistance since chronic inflammation is a major contributing factor.

3. Improved Lipid Profile: IF may improve lipid metabolism by reducing triglycerides and increasing high-density lipoprotein (HDL) cholesterol. This provides even more proof of insulin sensitivity.

4. Gene Expression: Insulin sensitivity genes may be impacted by insulin flow factor (IF). Certain genes associated with better glucose regulation are activated, according to some study.

Weight Loss:

1. Metabolic Adaptation: Fasting causes a change in metabolism that promotes the body to use fat reserves as an energy source when food is scarce. People who do this lose weight.

2. Preservation of Lean Mass: IF appears to preserve lean muscle mass while promoting fat loss since it raises growth hormone during fasting periods.

3. Option for a Sustainable Lifestyle: IF is a more likely long-term solution for weight reduction than drastically calorie-restricted diets.

4. Psychological advantages: Since time-restricted eating schedules are typically easier to stick to than other diets that require

avoiding certain food categories, intermittent fasting (IF) may offer psychological advantages.

Practical Things to Bear in Mind:

1. Personalization: There is no one-size-fits-all solution to IF. It is important to adjust the eating and fasting schedules to fit your preferences and lifestyle.

2. Hydration: It's critical to keep your body well hydrated during fasting. Water, herbal teas, and black coffee are frequently allowed and can help control hunger.

3. Meals High in Nutrients: Focus on consuming meals high in nutrients to ensure you get the vitamins and minerals you require. You need to eat a balanced diet to make the most of your eating window.

4. Patient Progress: The results of IF may vary from person to person. You should be patient and persistent as it may take some time for your body to adjust and show noticeable improvements in weight and insulin sensitivity. Speak with a Medical Professional: If you take medication or have underlying medical concerns, consult a healthcare professional to ensure that IF is safe and appropriate for your specific situation.

Intermittent fasting is a sensible, scientifically proven method for boosting insulin sensitivity and encouraging weight loss. Its scientific foundation, applicability, and potential benefits make it a strong choice for improving metabolic health and achieving long-term weight control. It should be customized to each person's needs and applied with a firm understanding of its guiding principles, just like any other nutritional plan.

IF may not be the best option for everyone, even though it might be a smart tactic for improving insulin sensitivity and losing weight. Women who are pregnant or breastfeeding, persons with certain medical conditions, and those who have a history of eating disorders should see a healthcare professional before beginning an IF program.

Intermittent fasting is a thoughtful nutritional strategy that relies on the ideas of calorie and hormone management. It offers a sensible means of enhancing insulin sensitivity and promoting weight loss, while individual outcomes may vary. Like any diet, IF should be used with a full understanding of its principles and potential benefits. It is advisable that you see a healthcare practitioner to determine whether IF is suitable for your specific circumstances.

CHAPTER 14

MEAL PLANS & RECIPES

Meal Plans and Recipes: A Hands-on Guide to Nutritious Eating

Proper planning and preparation of meals is essential for leading a healthier lifestyle. It's a rational, fact-based approach to eating that builds on the blending of tastes and nutrients. This in-depth manual will explore the nuances of meal planning and dish development, providing a rational, useful, and thorough synopsis.

I. Why Meal Planning Is Important

Achieving a well-rounded nutritional balance is the cornerstone of every effective meal plan. Think about the variety of micronutrients that, in addition to the three macronutrients—lipids, proteins, and carbohydrates—your body need.

Portion Control: A carefully considered meal plan considers what kinds and quantities of food are appropriate. Maintaining a healthy weight and preventing overindulgence require portion management.

The secret to success is consistency. Making regular eating decisions is facilitated by a well-thought-out meal plan, which supports long-term health advantages.

2. Establishing a Menu

Choose Your Objectives: Make a list of your dietary objectives first. Which would you prefer: maintaining your present weight or putting on more muscle? Your needs for calories and nutrients will depend on your goals.

Give whole foods a chance and choose for them instead of processed stuff. They offer a consistent source of energy and are high in minerals and fiber.

Balanced Macronutrients: Take your goals and nutritional requirements into account when determining your daily intake of fat, protein, and carbohydrates. Lean protein (chicken, tofu), complex carbs (quinoa, brown rice), and healthy fats (olive oil, avocado) are a few examples of foods that might be included in a balanced diet.

Foods that are adaptable: To get a variety of nutrients, change up your food. Include whole grains, lean proteins, veggies in your diet and fruits.

III. Choosing a Recipe Book
Variety and Flavor: Meal planning that is logical need not be boring. To spice up your dishes and add some excitement, try experimenting with different herbs and spices.

Simplicity: Not every dish has to be incredibly complex. Even simple meals may be delightful and satisfying. An omelet with feta and spinach, for instance, is a quick, nutrient-dense lunch that pairs nicely with a side of mixed berries.

Methods of Preparation: Grilling, roasting, and steaming are better options since they hold onto more nutrients than frying.

IV. Real-Life Case Studies

Breakfast-wise, overnight oats make sense. These are rolled oats soaked in yogurt and topped with nuts and berries. It has lots of fiber, protein, and good fats.

A substantial plate of grilled chicken salad topped with cucumbers, cherry tomatoes, and mixed greens with vinaigrette dressing would constitute lunch. This offers a variety of vitamins and minerals along with a balance of macronutrients.

Dinner is a simple yet nutritious meal that might be baked salmon, steamed broccoli, and quinoa. It provides a great source of protein, complex carbohydrates, and essential omega-3 fatty acids.

V. Being Reliability

Meal planning and ingredient preparation should be done in advance. This lessens the desire to choose rash, risky treatments.

Monitor Your Progress: Record your meals in a journal to assess how well you're adhering to the plan. In the long term, this could assist you in making the required changes.

Flexibility: Adapt to the limitations of your nutrition plan. It's acceptable to indulge sometimes as long as it doesn't impair your overall development.

VI. Reflective Snacks

Pick healthy snacks like carrot sticks with hummus or Greek yogurt with honey and nuts. Without the unnecessary calories seen in many processed meals, they offer vital nutrients.

Portion control is important, especially while eating healthy snacks. Serving sizes might help you overcome your compulsive overindulgence in food.

VII. Water's Significance

Water: It's easy to overlook the importance of maintaining proper hydration for general health. Water is necessary for digestion, energy production, and even hunger regulation. Make it a goal to drink eight glasses of water a day, or around two liters.

Herbal Teas: Drinking enticing, low-calorie herbal teas, such chamomile or green tea, may motivate you to consume more water.

VIII. Specific Nutritional Guidelines and Suggestions

Vegans and vegetarians: If you eat only plant-based foods, be sure to include a range of plant protein sources in your diet, such as beans, lentils, and tofu. Include fortified foods in your diet to fulfill your vitamin requirements, including B12.

Allergies and Intolerances: If you have any dietary allergies or intolerances, proceed with caution when reading labels and selecting appropriate replacements. To guarantee that your meal plan is both enjoyable and safe, there are a ton of allergen-free recipes available online.

IX. Tools for Meal Planning

apps: Create grocery lists, plan meals, and monitor your progress with the aid of meal planning websites and applications.

Cookbooks and Internet sites: There are a plethora of cookbooks and internet sites that offer a large selection of recipes to suit various dietary requirements and tastes.

X. Getting Used to the Change

Modifications to your way of life: Your diet should be modified appropriately. Adjust the number of calories you consume based on how active or inactive you are.

Health Conditions: If your condition changes, go to a trained nutritionist or healthcare provider and have your diet plan modified.

XI. Support and Community

Share Your Journey: If relatives or friends can act as a source of accountability and support, you might want to think about sharing your meal plan with them.

Seek Professional Advice: For individualized advice if you have any particular dietary requirements or health issues, see a licensed dietician.

XII. The Broadened Angle

Sustainability: A nutritious diet needs to be sustainable throughout time. Making long-term, healthy decisions is more important than looking for fast solutions.

To eat mindfully, concentrate on enjoying your food and pay attention to your body's signals of hunger and fullness.

Choosing recipes and organizing meals is a dynamic, lifelong activity that may encourage improved physical health as well as a stronger bond with food. You may enjoy a range of delectable meals and meet your nutritional and health objectives by adhering to a wise plan and practicing balanced eating. Never forget that every decision you make on a daily basis, no matter how tiny, has a big impact on your success.

To meet your nutritional objectives, meal planning and recipes are crucial tools. You may still enjoy a variety of flavors and make sure your body is getting the nutrients it needs by applying a methodical and scientific approach. To begin your journey toward better health and wellbeing, make sure your meals are wholesome and well-balanced, and carefully evaluate your objectives.